It's easy to
get lost in the
cancer world

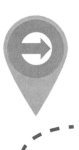

Let
**NCCN Guidelines
for Patients®
be your guide**

✓ Step-by-step guides to the cancer care options likely to have the best results

✓ Based on treatment guidelines used by health care providers worldwide

✓ Designed to help you discuss cancer treatment with your doctors

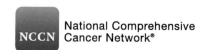

NCCN Guidelines for Patients® are developed by the National Comprehensive Cancer Network® (NCCN®)

NCCN

✓ An alliance of leading cancer centers across the United States devoted to patient care, research, and education

Cancer centers that are part of NCCN:
NCCN.org/cancercenters

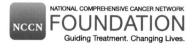

NCCN Clinical Practice Guidelines in Oncology (NCCN Guidelines®)

✓ Developed by doctors from NCCN cancer centers using the latest research and years of experience

✓ For providers of cancer care all over the world

✓ Expert recommendations for cancer screening, diagnosis, and treatment

Free online at
NCCN.org/guidelines

NCCN Guidelines for Patients

✓ Present information from the NCCN Guidelines in an easy-to-learn format

✓ For people with cancer and those who support them

✓ Explain the cancer care options likely to have the best results

Free online at
NCCN.org/patientguidelines

and supported by funding from NCCN Foundation®

These NCCN Guidelines for Patients are based on the NCCN Guidelines® for Distress Management (Version 2.2020, March 11, 2020).

NCCN Foundation seeks to support the millions of patients and their families affected by a cancer diagnosis by funding and distributing NCCN Guidelines for Patients. NCCN Foundation is also committed to advancing cancer treatment by funding the nation's promising doctors at the center of innovation in cancer research. For more details and the full library of patient and caregiver resources, visit NCCN.org/patients.

National Comprehensive Cancer Network (NCCN) / NCCN Foundation
3025 Chemical Road, Suite 100
Plymouth Meeting, PA 19462
215.690.0300

Sponsored by

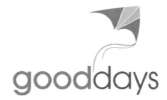

Good Days

Good Days is proud to support this educational resource for patients and their families and offers unwavering commitment to those who struggle with chronic disease, cancer, and other life-altering conditions. mygooddays.org

Endorsed by

American Psychosocial Oncology Society

American Psychosocial Oncology Society (APOS) is pleased to endorse the NCCN Guidelines for Patients: Distress During Cancer Care. APOS stands behind early psychosocial distress screening and distress management of cancer patients as an integral part of comprehensive cancer care. Education about distress management for those affected by cancer and all who support them will prove most valuable throughout the cancer journey. The NCCN Patient Guidelines provide this resource in an easily navigated document.
apos-society.org

Be the Match®

National Marrow Donor Program® (NMDP)/Be The Match® is the global leader in providing a possible cure to patients with life-threatening blood and marrow cancers, as well as other diseases. Our Be The Match Patient Support Center provides support, information, and resources for patients, caregivers, and families.
BeTheMatch.org/one-on-one

The Leukemia & Lymphoma Society

The Leukemia & Lymphoma Society (LLS) is dedicated to developing better outcomes for blood cancer patients and their families through research, education, support and advocacy and is happy to have this comprehensive resource available to patients.
lls.org/informationspecialists

To make a gift or learn more, please visit NCCNFoundation.org/donate or e-mail PatientGuidelines@nccn.org.

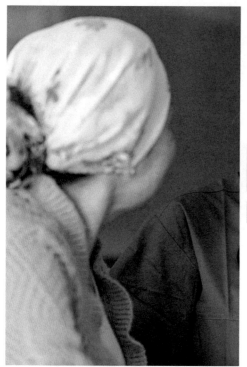

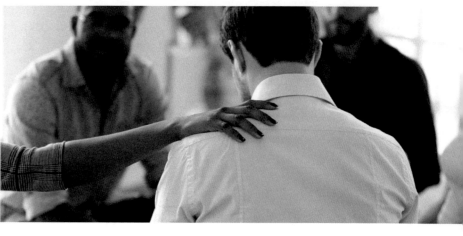

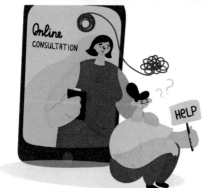

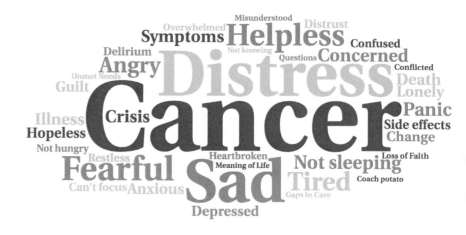

Misunderstood
Overwhelmed Distrust
Symptoms Helpless Confused
Delirium Not knowing Questions Concerned
Angry Distress Conflicted
Unmet Needs Death
Guilt Lonely
Illness Crisis Cancer Panic
Hopeless Side effects
Not hungry Change
Restless Heartbroken Loss of Faith
Fearful Meaning of Life Not sleeping
Can't focus Anxious Sad Tired Coach potato
Gaps in Care
Depressed

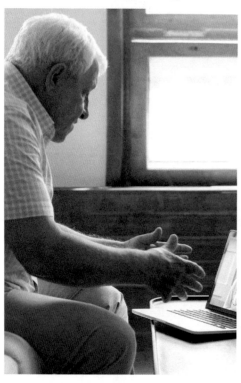

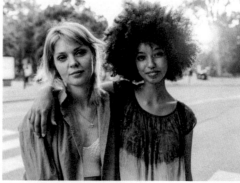

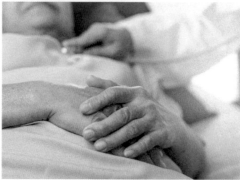

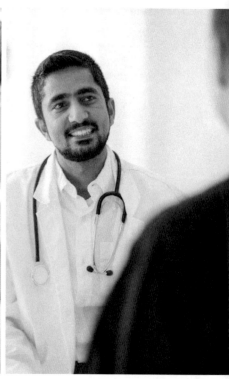

Contents

1
About distress

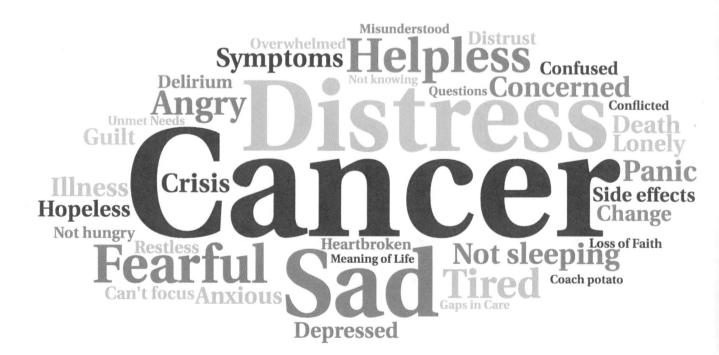

Everyone with cancer has some distress at some point in time. Distress is normal. Read this chapter to learn about the symptoms of distress and when distress is likely to occur.

Distress symptoms

Distress is an unpleasant experience of a mental, physical, social, or spiritual nature. It can affect the way you think, feel, or act. Distress is normal during cancer care, but it may make it harder to cope with cancer.

Distress ranges from mild to extreme levels. It can consist of common feelings like sadness, fear, and helplessness. Higher levels of distress can cause problems in one or more areas of life. It can affect a person's self-care, social life, mood, or faith.

Everyone with cancer has some distress at some point in time. It is normal to feel sad, fearful, and helpless. Distress is to be expected.

There are many symptoms of distress. Distress symptoms differ between people. They can change over time. Some symptoms of distress are listed in Guide 1.

Some symptoms of distress have other causes, too. An example is poor sleep. Poor sleep may be related to one or more factors, such as pain, heartburn, and medication.

Guide 1
Examples of distress symptoms
Sadness
Fear, worry, helplessness
Anger, feeling out of control
Concerns about illness and treatment
Worries about paying bills and costs of living
Questioning your faith, your purpose, the meaning of life
Pulling away from too many people
Concerns about taking care of others, such as a child or parent
Poor sleep, appetite, or concentration
Depression, anxiety, panic
Frequent thoughts of illness or death

You just can't imagine how much fear and anxiety builds up.

– Dan
  Survivor, Non-Small Cell Lung Cancer

Causes and risk factors

There isn't just one cause of distress. The cause of distress differs between people. For example, some people may be distressed from having severe side effects from treatment. Other people may be distressed from the amount of money needed to pay their bills. Even if you have been wise with your money, the costs related to cancer can add up.

Anyone can become distressed, but some people are more likely to than others. A risk factor is anything that increases the chance of an event. There is a wide range of risk factors for distress. Some of these risk factors are listed in Guide 2.

Health-related factors

People with uncontrolled symptoms are more likely to be distressed. Some people have symptoms from the cancer, from the cancer treatment, or both. If symptoms are severe or long-lasting, the chance of becoming distressed increases.

Certain medical conditions can lead to distress. An example is having cancer and another severe illness. Having cognitive impairment, like poor memory, may make dealing with cancer very hard. Another example is the link between depression and some cancers, such as pancreatic and head and neck cancers.

Access to care

Having limited access to health care can also lead to distress. Some people may not have health insurance or not enough insurance. Others may need to travel far to see a health provider. Some people have a hard time finding a health provider who meets their needs.

Guide 2
Risk factors for distress

Distress is more likely in people who:

Have uncontrolled symptoms

Have a severe illness in addition to cancer

Have cognitive impairment

Have a cancer that is linked to depression

Have limited access to health care

Have money problems

Are younger in age

Have spiritual or religious concerns

Are unable to communicate as needed

Have family conflicts

Lack social support

Live alone

Live in a new country (immigration)

Don't have a stable place to live

Have younger or dependent children

Have suffered trauma like physical or sexual abuse

Have attempted suicide

Have had a substance use disorder or are currently misusing alcohol or drugs

Have had a mental disorder like major depression or generalized anxiety disorder

Financial factors

Money may get even tighter during cancer care. There may be less money due to travel costs, insurance co-payments, and missing work. With less money, the chance of becoming distressed increases.

Personal factors

Personal risk factors for distress include being young. Younger people may be very shocked to learn that they have cancer. It may be too much to deal with cancer and everyday life.

Some people have concerns related to their religious faith or spirituality. Their concerns may be long-standing or new. These concerns put people at risk for being distressed.

Social factors

Distress is more likely when there are problems with communication. Health providers may use words that their patients don't know. Some people with cancer have trouble expressing their needs. Contacting health providers may not be easy.

Family conflict, lack of support, or living alone may increase the burden of having cancer. Unstable housing or the challenges of immigration may add to stress.

Children are an important responsibility. Caring for children while dealing with cancer can be very hard. People with cancer who care for children are more likely to be distressed.

Mental health factors

Poor mental health before cancer is linked to distress after cancer. Past trauma can affect mental well-being. It increases the risk for distress during cancer care. Trauma includes physical, sexual, verbal, or emotional abuse.

A past suicide attempt is linked to distress among people with cancer. Suicide can stem from deep feelings of hopelessness. These feelings may resurface during cancer care.

People who have had a mental health disorder (or mental illness) are more likely to be distressed during cancer care. Common mental health disorders include substance use disorders, mood disorders, and anxiety disorders.

> ❯ Substance use disorders are defined by problems caused by the use of alcohol or drugs.

> ❯ Symptoms of mood disorders are depression, mania, or both.

> ❯ Symptoms of anxiety disorders are ongoing and intense worry, fear, or panic.

On a daily basis, I come across patients who are being absolutely drained of the resources they need.

– Dr. Fahd
Oncologist

Triggers

Distress can occur at any point in time. However, there are times when being distressed is more likely. Guide 3 includes a list of times when distress is more likely.

Testing
You may become distressed when getting tested. An example is being distressed when getting tests for a symptom or lump. After getting tested, you may need to wait for the results. Waiting for test results can be hard.

The first response to learning of a cancer diagnosis is often shock. You may also be worried, fearful, or sad. Further testing may be needed to learn more about the cancer you have.

When cancer appears cured or well-controlled, people get tests on a regular basis. Going to check-up visits and waiting for test results can be stressful. Distress is common if the cancer returns or worsens.

Treatment
Waiting for treatment to start can trigger distress. Cancer treatment may cause distressing health problems (that is, complications and side effects). Distress is also common after learning that treatment didn't work.

Transitions in care
Transitions in care can also lead to distress. Examples of a transition include being discharged from the hospital or finishing all treatment. Shifting from frequent treatment visits to less frequent follow-up visits is a big change.

Guide 3
Triggers of distress

Distress is likely to start or worsen when:

A new symptom prompts testing

Being tested for cancer

Learning the diagnosis

Learning the cancer is advanced

Learning you have a genetic risk for cancer

Waiting for treatment to start

Symptoms get worse

Having a treatment-related complication

Being admitted to or discharged from a hospital

Starting another type of treatment

Learning that treatment didn't work

Finishing treatment

Receiving follow-up care and cancer tests

Learning the cancer returned or worsened

Starting end-of-life care

Impact on life

In this section, some of the negative effects of distress are described. These negative effects show why distress screening and treatment are so important.

By definition, being distressed isn't pleasant. Feeling distressed doesn't make coping with cancer any easier. You are stressed enough with learning about cancer, getting cancer care, and doing your everyday duties.

Distress may affect how well you function. Distress can interfere with sleep. You might sleep less or more than normal. Distress may lessen your ability to focus. You may need to ask people to repeat what they said because you lost track. Distress may affect how well you relate to people. You may pull away from others. If you have children, you may have trouble taking care of them.

Distress may interfere with your health decisions or actions. People who are distressed are less likely to take their medicines as their doctor prescribed. They may also have trouble making treatment decisions and be less likely to exercise and quit smoking.

Distressed people are also less likely to go to follow-up visits. This can lead to health problems followed by even more visits to the doctor's office and emergency room.

Distress may worsen your health. Distress leads to poorer quality of life. It may even have a harmful impact on your length of life.

Poor mental health can further worsen from distress during cancer care. At high levels, distress can result in a mental health disorder.

Review

> Distress is normal, common, and expected. Common symptoms are sadness, fear, and helplessness.

> Distress ranges from mild to extreme levels. Everyone with cancer has some level of distress at some point in time.

> Some people are more likely to be distressed than others. People who have uncontrolled symptoms, money problems, lack of support, or a history of mental illness are likely to be distressed.

> There will be times when being distressed is more likely. A change in your health, treatment, or health providers can trigger distress. Distress is common after learning the cancer has returned or worsened.

> Being distressed makes it harder to cope with cancer. It can limit how well you function. Distress can also lead to worse physical and mental health.

It's hard to deal with all of the things that happen at once, and not to just collapse and worry and stress.

— Pauline
  Wife of a Cancer Survivor

2
Distress screening

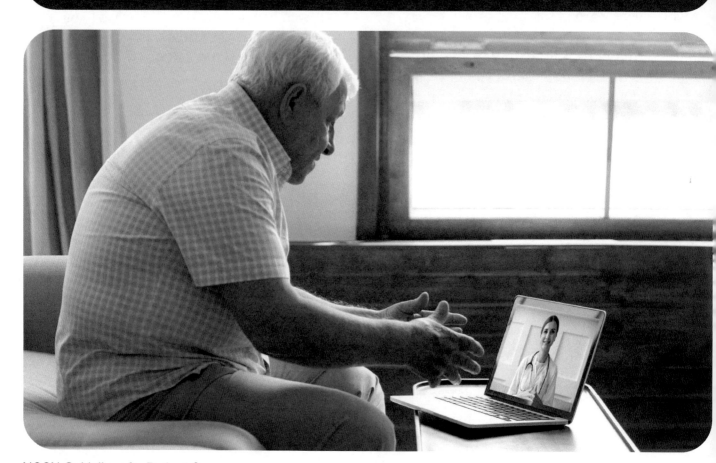

Assessing distress is a key part of cancer care. This chapter describes the screening process for distress and who can help you. Distress screening, when paired with getting help, improves lives.

Screening tools

A screening tool is a short assessment for a condition. For distress, screening tools prompt you to respond to one or more statements or questions. Screening tools are often paper-based but are also given via hand-held smart devices, interactive voice responses, and internet-based programs.

Distress screening tools have been tested in research studies. They have been found to work well for detecting who is distressed and pinpointing people's needs.

NCCN Distress Thermometer and Problem List

The NCCN Distress Thermometer and Problem List is a well-known screening tool among cancer care providers. It has been shown in many studies to work well.

The Distress Thermometer measures distress on a 0 to 10 scale. To report your distress, circle the number that matches your level of distress in the past week.

The Problem List includes problems from 5 areas of life: practical, family, emotional, spiritual/religious, and physical problems. The Problem List can be changed to fit the hardships of a particular group of people.

The Problem List will help your cancer care team learn what is causing your distress. Your team will ask better follow-up questions. You will be referred to the right help if needed.

Ideally, you would be screened for distress at every health care visit. You should be screened for distress at time points when distress is likely (for example, at diagnosis). If you aren't screened for distress at appointments, you can show your team your responses to the NCCN Distress Thermometer and Problem List that are on the next page.

I talk with people every day who are in a place of despair. When they call us, they've usually just experienced a one-two punch. First, they've been told they have cancer. Second, after receiving encouraging news that there is medication that can potentially save their lives, they are devastated to discover the out-of-pocket cost of the medication is beyond their financial means, because insurance won't pay the full amount.

– Fran
Patient Care Specialist

NCCN Distress Thermometer

Distress is an unpleasant experience of a mental, physical, social, or spiritual nature. It can affect the way you think, feel, or act. Distress may make it harder to cope with having cancer, its symptoms, or its treatment.

Instructions: Please circle the number (0–10) that best describes how much distress you have been experiencing in the past week including today.

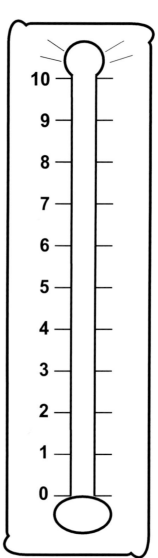

Extreme distress — 10

No distress — 0

Problem List

Please indicate if any of the following has been a problem for you in the past week including today. Be sure to check **Yes** or **No** for each.

Yes	No	**Practical Problems**	Yes	No	**Physical Problems**
❑	❑	Child care	❑	❑	Appearance
❑	❑	Food	❑	❑	Bathing/dressing
❑	❑	Housing	❑	❑	Breathing
❑	❑	Insurance/financial	❑	❑	Changes in urination
❑	❑	Transportation	❑	❑	Constipation
❑	❑	Work/school	❑	❑	Diarrhea
❑	❑	Treatment decisions	❑	❑	Eating
			❑	❑	Fatigue
		Family Problems	❑	❑	Feeling swollen
❑	❑	Dealing with children	❑	❑	Fevers
❑	❑	Dealing with partner	❑	❑	Getting around
❑	❑	Ability to have children	❑	❑	Indigestion
❑	❑	Family health issues	❑	❑	Memory/concentration
			❑	❑	Mouth sores
		Emotional Problems	❑	❑	Nausea
❑	❑	Depression	❑	❑	Nose dry/congested
❑	❑	Fears	❑	❑	Pain
❑	❑	Nervousness	❑	❑	Sexual
❑	❑	Sadness	❑	❑	Skin dry/itchy
❑	❑	Worry	❑	❑	Sleep
❑	❑	Loss of interest in usual activities	❑	❑	Substance use
			❑	❑	Tingling in hands/feet

❑ ❑ **Spiritual/religious concerns**

Other Problems:_____

_____

Screening results

Distress screening is usually fast. A member of your cancer care team will discuss the results with you. Your results will be used to get you the help you need.

Some types of distress may be managed by your cancer care team. Your team has a wide range of knowledge and skills. For some types of distress, they may refer you to people with a different set of knowledge and skills. After you complete a screener of distress, a member of your team may:

> Assess your distress further

> Treat ongoing physical symptoms

> Manage mild distress symptoms

> Refer you to experts in distress

Referral to experts

There are providers who have completed special training for treating distress. Your cancer care team may refer you to one or more of these experts based on your screening results. In this section, some of the experts in distress are described. Their qualifications and the issues they treat are explained.

Chaplains

You may mark on a screening tool that you have spiritual or religious concerns. Many cancer centers have a chaplain on staff. If not, your cancer care team will likely know of one in the community. Many distressed people are interested in meeting with a chaplain.

Many chaplains are certified and have finished a specific course of training to provide chaplaincy services. They are certified as either board-certified chaplains or associate certified chaplains.

Chaplains help people of any faith or no faith. They provide care for issues like:

> Conflict between people over beliefs

> Conflicts between beliefs and treatment

> Concerns or needs relating to faith, purpose, or meaning of life

> Concerns about dying or the afterlife

> Grief, guilt, and forgiveness

> Loneliness and self-worth

Hope is a huge part of the cancer process. Because, if you lose that, you don't have the inner strength you need to fight.

– Kris
Survivor, Multiple Myeloma

Social workers

Social workers help people cope with life challenges. They have earned either a bachelor's or master's degree in social work. Some go on to earn a doctoral degree.

Social workers can choose a specific area of practice. Oncology social workers provide a range of services to the cancer community. Clinical social workers are mental health professionals. They must obtain a state license to practice.

Social workers provide help for practical and psychosocial problems, such as:

> Housing, food, and transportation

> Insurance and bills

> Assistance with self-care and dependent care

> Treatment decisions and advance directives

> Grief, loss, and adjusting to changes in one's health and body

> Anxiety, trauma, depression, and thoughts of suicide

> Family, social, and cultural issues

Psychologists

Psychologists are mental health professionals. Most psychologists have a doctoral degree in psychology. The two doctoral degrees that can be earned are a PhD and PsyD in psychology. All psychologists complete an internship. Some psychologists pursue more training in a post-doctoral fellowship, obtain board certification, or both.

There are different fields of psychology. Psychologists who provide clinical services include clinical psychologists, counseling psychologists, health psychologists, neuropsychologists, and school psychologists. A state license is required to provide clinical services. In some states, psychologists can prescribe medications for mental health after obtaining the proper education, training, and state certification.

Depending on their training, psychologists provide treatment for the following:

> Health issues, such as pain, weight, sleep, sex, and taking medications as prescribed

> Cognitive problems, such as dementia and chemo brain

> Mood and anxiety problems, such as depression, panic, and worry

> Substance use, such as drugs, alcohol, and smoking

> Thoughts of suicide

> Relationship issues, such as caregiving strains and social conflicts

Psychiatrists

Psychiatrists are medical doctors who specialize in mental health. They are experts in how the body and mind affect each other. They are able to assess both physical and mental health.

Psychiatrists have either an MD or DO degree. They obtain a state license to practice and complete a residency program in psychiatry. Most become board-certified in psychiatry.

Psychiatrists can obtain more training and become certified in a particular area. These areas include child and adolescent psychiatry, geriatric psychiatry, addiction psychiatry, and consultation-liaison psychiatry. Some consultation-liaison psychiatrists specialize in working with cancer patients.

Psychiatrists are trained to treat mental, emotional, and addictive disorders. Some of the common disorders treated by psychiatrists include depression, general anxiety, bipolar, panic, psychotic, eating, and substance use disorders. Psychiatrists may be particularly helpful when mental disorders:

> Are hard to diagnose,

> Occur with physical conditions,

> Require medication to manage,

> Need treatment in a hospital,

> Occur suddenly or over a long period of time, or

> Are not responding to standard treatment.

Nurses

There are many types of nurses who care for people with cancer. A registered nurse (RN) is the most common type. RNs have earned at least an Associate's degree or a diploma from a hospital-based program. They need a state license to practice. Some RNs go on to earn a master's or doctoral degree in nursing.

Another type of nurse is an advanced practice registered nurse (APRN). An APRN is an RN who has earned at least a master's degree in nursing. There are four types of APRNs: nurse practitioner (NP), clinical nurse specialist (CNS), certified nurse anesthetist, and certified nurse midwife. An APRN state license is needed to practice. APRNs can prescribe medication.

Nurses can also obtain certification in specialty areas. Examples of certification include oncology and psychiatry. Oncology nurses provide a high quality of care to people with cancer. Psychiatric nurses are mental health experts.

Nurses are on the front line of cancer care. They are often the first to detect that a person is distressed. They may be the one to screen you for distress. Across the many types of nursing, nurses provide help for a wide range of problems related to distress, such as:

> Practical matters like needing a ride to appointments

> Lack of knowledge about cancer

> Physical symptoms and illnesses

> Complex health care systems

> Mental health symptoms and disorders

Benefits of screening

If paired with getting help, distress screening can yield major benefits. Some of the benefits of distress screening are listed next.

Detects people in distress

Without standard screening, many distressed people are not identified and don't get the help they need. Often, doctors don't ask, and patients don't tell their doctors about their distress. Screening tools empower doctors to ask about distress. They also empower people with cancer to share how they are feeling.

In-depth evaluation

You may receive an in-depth evaluation depending on what is distressing you. An example is memory testing if you say your memory is a big problem. Another example is a clinical assessment for high distress about sexual problems or pain. A clinical assessment may include:

> - An interview
> - Survey
> - Health or brain function tests

Better distress management

Early distress screening leads to timely management of distress. A study of routine screening showed that distressed people who were referred for help were less distressed 3 months later. Better management of distress in turn improves self-care and health outcomes.

Improved self-care

Treating distress makes it easier to stay on track with cancer treatment. You will be less likely to miss doctor's visits and skip taking your medicines. You will likely need to contact your doctor less often. When not distressed, communication with your treatment team will be easier and better.

Improved health outcomes

Treating distress early helps to prevent emotional problems from becoming severe. If distress is treated, you likely won't be angry all the time or be intensely angry. Severe anxiety and depression may also be avoided. In addition to better mental health, treating distress improves health-related quality of life and may help your physical health.

Review

> - A screening tool for distress is a brief survey of your perceived distress.

> - The NCCN Distress Thermometer and Problem List were created by NCCN experts to assess the level and nature of your distress.

> - Your cancer care team will treat mild distress or refer you to experts in distress.

> - Experts in distress have obtained education, training, and credentials to conduct evaluations and provide treatment. Depending on your needs, you may be referred to a chaplain, social worker, psychologist, psychiatrist, psychiatric nurse, or another mental health provider.

> - Distress screening that is paired with getting help can improve well-being and health.

3
Treatment for distress

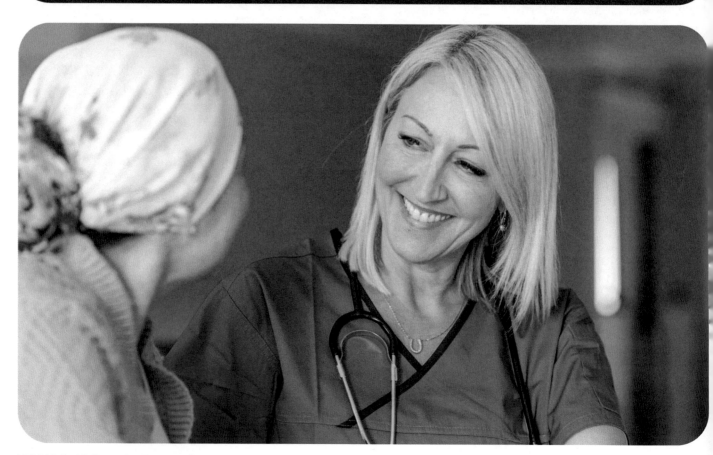

There is a wide range of help for distress. This chapter is an overview of the common types of help for people with cancer.

Cancer care team

The cancer care team often manages mild distress. Mild distress is also called expected distress. It includes worry about the future and concerns about treatment. Your team can manage mild distress by:

> Explaining distress is normal and what to expect

> Providing education on cancer and its treatment

> Discussing advance care planning

> Prescribing medication

> Preventing gaps in care between health care providers

> Teaching new or better ways to cope

> Sharing information about resources at your cancer center and in your community

Cancer education

Having cancer is very stressful. One stressor is the need to learn about cancer care. Your care team can answer questions and direct you to trusted educational resources. Learning from trusted educational resources can be very helpful and reduce stress.

There may be a learning center at your cancer center. The learning center may have printed materials or have access to online resources. Health educators can help you find trusted information.

Your cancer center may have a patient navigator program. Patient navigators educate. They can explain your plan of care. They can tell you what to expect at appointments and from treatment. They can give you educational materials.

NCCN has a growing library of NCCN Guidelines for Patients®. These resources are a good starting point from which to learn the best options for cancer care. Your cancer care team can provide more information to help you make treatment decisions. Visit NCCN.org/patients for resources on cancer screening, cancer treatment, and supportive care.

Chaplaincy care

Many people with cancer find spirituality or religion helpful. People use spiritual or religious resources to cope with cancer. Receiving spiritual support may improve quality of life and satisfaction with care.

A chaplain can help whether you have strong beliefs, different beliefs, conflicted beliefs, or no beliefs. Chaplains provide a range of services including:

> Spiritual or existential support to foster peace and comfort

> Counseling in line with your faith or beliefs

> Guidance to discover spirituality or purpose

> Prayer

> Guided meditation

> Spiritual or religious rituals

> Liaison between patients and spiritual communities

> Referral to health care providers

Social work and counseling services

Social workers provide services for practical or psychosocial problems. Patient navigators and case managers may be of help, too. Practical problems commonly relate to illness, food, money, work, school, language, and caregiving. Psychosocial problems include mental and social effects of the cancer.

People with practical and psychosocial problems are often helped by social work and counseling services. Otherwise, some of these problems may be addressed by mental health services, which are described in the next section. Social workers address practical and psychosocial problems by:

> Connecting patients to resources

> Advocating on behalf of patients

> Teaching patients and families

> Leading support groups

> Counseling patients, couples, and families

> Contacting protective services

> Giving a referral to a mental health provider

> Giving a referral to a chaplain

I worried how we would survive this financially.

– Carol
Survivor, Multiple Myeloma

Mental health services

There are many types of mental health providers. Examples include clinical social workers, psychologists, advanced practice clinicians, psychiatric nurses, and psychiatrists. The work of these providers overlaps, but their expertise varies. You should be referred to a provider who is a good fit for your needs.

Evaluation

The first step of care is often an evaluation to assess the problem. Evaluations differ between people based on the type of distress. You may be evaluated for:

- Changes in behavior
- Pain, fatigue, or lack of sleep
- Sexual health
- Current and past mental health
- Treatment history
- Medical causes
- Alcohol and drug use
- Cognitive problems
- Body image
- Suicidal thoughts and plan
- Safety

Treatment

There are many types of mental health treatment. Based on the evaluation, your provider will make a treatment plan tailored to you. Mental health treatment works well to reduce distress and improve quality of life among people with cancer.

Counseling and psychotherapy

Some people think of psychotherapy and counseling as the same thing. Both help people feel better, solve problems, and achieve life goals. Both are sometimes called "talk therapy."

Many providers think of them as two distinct treatments. Counseling is often thought as short-term help for outward behaviors. In contrast, psychotherapy is in-depth, sometimes long-term, help that addresses the inner person. The differences between the two treatments have lessened over time.

Counseling often focuses on a specific issue. Examples include adjusting to illness, grief, and stress management. The methods used in counseling vary based on the issue.

Psychotherapy can help with a broad range of mental health needs. Cognitive behavioral therapy (CBT) focuses on changing thoughts and actions that contribute to poor mental health. It can help with depression, anxiety, pain, and fatigue among people with cancer.

Supportive psychotherapy uses a flexible approach to meet people's changing needs. It is widely used to help people with cancer. Sub-types of this psychotherapy include supportive-expressive, cognitive-existential, and meaning-centered psychotherapy.

Types of mental health treatment include:

> Watchful waiting on level of distress

> Education on mental health issues

> Psychotherapy or counseling; also called "talk therapy"

> Cognitive rehabilitation to improve brain functioning

> Behavioral management

> Suicide prevention

> Psychiatric medication

> Medications for drug detoxification and to prevent relapse

> Electroconvulsive therapy

> Hospital care, residential treatment, and specialized programs

> Exercise

> Integrative (or complementary) therapy like yoga or meditation

Psychiatric medications

Psychiatric (or psychotropic) medications are drugs that improve mental health. Psychiatric medications are grouped by how they are commonly used.

Antidepressants are commonly used to treat depression. Two key features of depression are: 1) feeling down or irritable; and 2) losing interest in things that you used to like. Antidepressants are also used to treat anxiety and certain physical problems like pain.

Anxiolytics may be used with psychotherapy to treat anxiety. Key features of anxiety include severe fear or worry, panic attacks, and strong behavioral impulses.

Mood stabilizers treat bipolar-related disorders. The key feature of bipolar disorders is an episode of elevated mood called mania.

Antipsychotics treat psychotic disorders. Features of psychotic disorders include perceiving unreal sensations, fixed false beliefs, and disorganized thinking.

Antipsychotics treat other health conditions, too. They may be used to treat anxiety if other medications did not work. Antipsychotics are also used to treat delirium—a short-term disturbance in mental abilities. Delirium occurs in people with advanced cancer. It can also be triggered by some types of medicines.

Review

- The cancer care team often treats mild distress.

- A chaplain can help people of any faith or no faith. Chaplains provide support, counseling, and guidance to people in need.

- Social workers provide help for practical or psychosocial problems. These problems may be relieved by learning new information or skills, counseling, attending support groups, or community resources.

- Mental health providers perform evaluations to inform treatment planning. Common mental health services include education, psychotherapy, and prescribing medications.

Initially, you're doing everything you can to survive. You can kind of get used to that. You're constantly fighting. Then, after a while, you get a chance to pop your head above water for a little bit and look around. You see all the people who are trying to throw you flotation. People trying to help you keep your head above water and not sink. People yelling out words of encouragement to you. And so ... you keep going.

– Steve
  Brother of a Cancer Survivor

4
Getting help

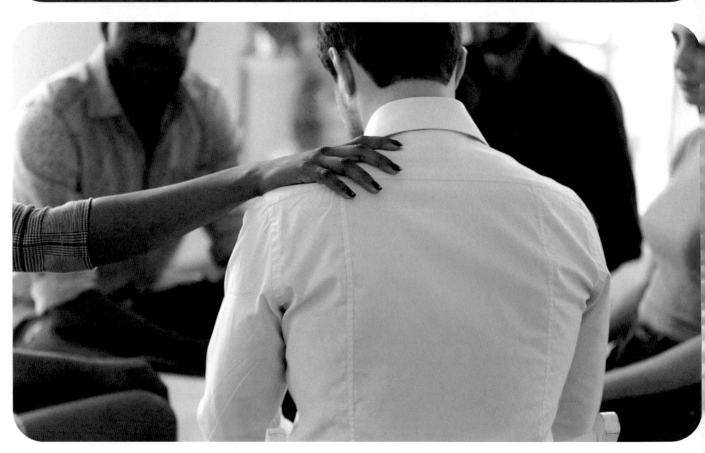

Every distressed person with cancer should receive help. This chapter gives a history of how distress management has become a standard of cancer care. It also provides a list of questions and websites for you to use.

Standard of care

Everyone with cancer has some distress at some point in time. However, distressed people with cancer have been underserved for decades. In 1997, NCCN made a groundbreaking step by forming a panel to develop treatment guidelines for distress. The first guidelines for distress were completed in 1999. This book is based on the most current version of the guidelines.

The National Academy of Medicine (NAM; formerly called the Institute of Medicine [IOM]) is a nonprofit group that provides advice to the United States. Its aim is to help people make good health decisions. The NAM is greatly respected among health care professionals.

In 2007, the IOM released a report called *Cancer Care for the Whole Patient*. In this report, a treatment model for distress was proposed. The model is based on the work of the NCCN Panel. It includes routine distress screening, treatment planning, referrals to experts in distress, and re-evaluation. The IOM report made distress management a new standard of quality cancer care.

The Commission on Cancer is a program of the American College of Surgeons. It grants accreditation to cancer centers that apply and meet their standards of quality cancer care.

In 2015, new standards went into effect for cancer centers. These new standards included distress screening.

This history is important to know. You should expect to receive distress screening and help at your cancer care visits. If your distress isn't addressed, ask for help.

Questions to ask

Ask your health care providers questions about distress. Being informed will help you make decisions. The questions on the next pages are in regard to the care you read about in this book. Feel free to use them or ask your own questions.

It may help to prepare questions before your visit. At the visit, repeat the answers given to you to confirm what you heard. You can also take notes. Many people bring their spouse, partner, friend, or other family member for support.

Questions to ask about distress

1. Is my symptom(s) part of being distressed?

2. Will my distress just go away in time?

3. How can you help me?

4. How can I help myself?

5. What help will my insurance cover?

_____

_____

_____

_____

_____

_____

_____

Questions to ask about cancer

1. What type of cancer do I have? Will it grow fast?

2. What tests do I need? How often are these tests wrong?

3. What options do I have? What will happen if I do nothing?

4. What are the pros and cons of each option? What are the side effects of treatment? What does each option require of me in terms of travel, time off, costs, and so forth?

5. What can be done to prevent or relieve side effects?

6. What are my chances that the cancer will return?

7. Are you board-certified? If yes, in what area? How many people like me have you treated?

Questions to ask about spiritual care

1. What do chaplains do?

2. Are chaplains ministers or priests?

3. Can a chaplain help me if we're not of the same faith or if I have no faith?

4. Can a chaplain help other family members?

Questions to ask about social work and counseling

1. What do social workers do?

2. Can you help me find a local support group?

3. Is there help for the high costs of cancer care?

4. Can you show me how to talk with my children, family, and friends?

5. How do I deal with people who are treating me differently?

6. How can counseling help with intimacy?

7. Can you help me get an advance directive?

Questions to ask about mental health services

1. What's the difference between the different types of mental health providers?

2. What's your expertise?

3. What are you testing me for? How long does testing take?

4. How will psychoeducation help me?

5. Will psychiatric medicine affect my cancer treatment? How long until the medicine works? What are the side effects of psychiatric medicine? How long do I need to take psychiatric medicine?

6. How does talk therapy help with distress? How do I choose a therapist?

7. Is there proof that complementary therapy or exercise helps distress?

Websites

Distress is to be expected when facing cancer. There are community resources that can help. Free online information can be found at the websites listed next.

Cancer information

Be the Match®
BeTheMatch.org/one-on-one

NCCN
MyCancerGuides.org

National Cancer Institute (NCI)
cancer.gov/resources-for/patients

The Leukemia & Lymphoma Society
lls.org/informationspecialists

Distress care

Alliance for Quality Psychosocial Cancer Care
wholecancerpatient.org

American Psychosocial Oncology Society
apos-society.org

Fertility

MyOncofertility.org
myoncofertility.org

NCCN
NCCN.org/patients

Spirituality

National Cancer Institute (NCI)
cancer.gov/cancertopics/pdq/supportivecare/spirituality/Patient

Support services

CancerCare
cancercare.org

Cancer Support Community
cancersupportcommunity.org

Good Days
mygooddays.org

National Coalition for Cancer Survivorship
canceradvocacy.org/resources/cancer-survival-toolbox

Review

> Distress management is a new standard of quality cancer care. Expect and ask for help from your cancer care team.

> Ask your health care providers questions about distress. Being informed will help you make decisions.

> There are community resources that can help. Many of these resources can be found online.

Words to know

APRN
Advanced practice registered nurse

CBT
Cognitive behavioral therapy

chaplain
A trained expert in providing spiritual care.

CNS
clinical nurse specialist

cognitive impairment
Trouble remembering, learning new things, concentrating, or making decisions that affect everyday life.

diagnosis
To identify a disease.

distress
An unpleasant experience of a mental, physical, social, or spiritual nature.

IOM
Institute of Medicine

oncologist
A medical doctor who's an expert in the treatment of cancer.

NAM
National Academy of Medicine

NCCN®
National Comprehensive Cancer Network®

NP
Nurse practitioner

RN
Registered nurse

psychiatrist
A medical doctor who's an expert in mental health.

psychologist
A trained expert in the human mind and behavior.

risk factor
Anything that increases the chance of an event.

screening tool
A short assessment for a condition.

side effect
An unplanned physical or emotional response to treatment.

social worker
An expert in meeting people's social and emotional needs.

substance use disorder
Repeated use of alcohol, drugs, or tobacco that causes major life problems.

NCCN Contributors

This patient guide is based on the NCCN Clinical Practice Guidelines in Oncology (NCCN Guidelines®) for Distress Management. It was adapted, reviewed, and published with help from the following people:

Dorothy A. Shead, MS
Director, Patient Information Operations

Laura J. Hanisch, PsyD
Medical Writer/Patient Information Specialist

Erin Vidic, MA
Medical Writer

Rachael Clarke
Senior Medical Copyeditor

Tanya Fischer, MEd, MSLIS
Medical Writer

Kim Williams
Creative Services Manager

Susan Kidney
Design Specialist

The NCCN Clinical Practice Guidelines in Oncology (NCCN Guidelines®) for Distress Management, Version 2.2020 were developed by the following NCCN Panel Members:

Michelle B. Riba, MD, MS/Chair
University of Michigan Rogel Cancer Center

Kristine A. Donovan, PhD, MBA/ Vice-Chair
Moffitt Cancer Center

Barbara Andersen, PhD
The Ohio State University Comprehensive Cancer Center - James Cancer Hospital and Solove Research Institute

Ilana Braun, MD
Dana-Farber/Brigham and Women's Cancer Center

William S. Breitbart, MD
Memorial Sloan Kettering Cancer Center

Benjamin W. Brewer, PsyD
University of Colorado Cancer Center

Luke O. Buchmann, MD
Huntsman Cancer Institute at the University of Utah

Molly Collins, MD
Fox Chase Cancer Center

Cheyenne Corbett, PhD
Duke Cancer Institute

Stewart Fleishman, MD
Consultant

Sofia Garcia, PhD
Robert H. Lurie Comprehensive Cancer Center of Northwestern University

Donna B. Greenberg, MD
Dana-Farber/Brigham and Women'sCancer Center| Massachusetts General Hospital Cancer Center

* **Rev. George F. Handzo, MA, MD**
Consultant

Laura Hoofring, MSN, APRN
The Sidney Kimmel Comprehensive Cancer Center at Johns Hopkins

Chao-Hui Huang, PhD
O'Neal Comprehensive Cancer Center at UAB

Pallavi Kumar, MD, MPH
Abramson Cancer Center at the University of Pennsylvania

Robin Lally, PhD, MS, RN
Fred & Pamela Buffett Cancer Center

Sara Martin, MD
Vanderbilt-Ingram Cancer Center

Lisa McGuffey, PhD, JD
University of Wisconsin Carbone Cancer Center

William Mitchell, MD
UC San Diego Moores Cancer Center

Laura J. Morrison, MD
Yale Cancer Center/Smilow Cancer Hospital

* **Shehzad K. Niazi, MD**
Mayo Clinic Cancer Center

Megan Pailler, PhD
Roswell Park Comprehensive Cancer Center

* **Oxana Palesh, PhD, MPH**
Stanford Cancer Institute

* **Francine Parnes, JD, MA**
Patient Advocate

Janice P. Pazar, RN, PhD
St. Jude Children's Research Hospital/ The University of Tennessee Health Science Center

Laurel Ralston, DO
Case Comprehensive Cancer Center/ University Hospitals Seidman Cancer Center and Cleveland Clinic Taussig Cancer Institute

Jaroslava Salman, MD
City of Hope National Medical Center

* **Moreen M. Shannon-Dudley, MSW**
Fred Hutchinson Cancer Research Center/ Seattle Cancer Care Alliance

Alan D. Valentine, MD
The University of Texas MD Anderson Cancer Center

Jessica Vanderlan, PhD
Siteman Cancer Center at Barnes- Jewish Hosptial and Washington University School of Medicine

NCCN Staff

Susan Darlow, PhD
Oncology Scientist, Medical Writer

Jennifer Keller, MSS
Guidelines Layout Specialist

Nicole McMillian, MS
Guidelines Coordinator

* Reviewed this patient guide. For disclosures, visit NCCN.org/about/disclosure.aspx.

NCCN Cancer Centers

Abramson Cancer Center
at the University of Pennsylvania
Philadelphia, Pennsylvania
800.789.7366 • pennmedicine.org/cancer

Fred & Pamela Buffett Cancer Center
Omaha, Nebraska
800.999.5465 • nebraskamed.com/cancer

Case Comprehensive Cancer Center/
University Hospitals Seidman Cancer
Center and Cleveland Clinic Taussig
Cancer Institute
Cleveland, Ohio
800.641.2422 • UH Seidman Cancer Center
uhhospitals.org/services/cancer-services
866.223.8100 • CC Taussig Cancer Institute
my.clevelandclinic.org/departments/cancer
216.844.8797 • Case CCC
case.edu/cancer

City of Hope National Medical Center
Los Angeles, California
800.826.4673 • cityofhope.org

Dana-Farber/Brigham and
Women's Cancer Center
Massachusetts General Hospital
Cancer Center
Boston, Massachusetts
877.332.4294
dfbwcc.org
massgeneral.org/cancer

Duke Cancer Institute
Durham, North Carolina
888.275.3853 • dukecancerinstitute.org

Fox Chase Cancer Center
Philadelphia, Pennsylvania
888.369.2427 • foxchase.org

Huntsman Cancer Institute
at the University of Utah
Salt Lake City, Utah
877.585.0303
huntsmancancer.org

Fred Hutchinson Cancer
Research Center/Seattle
Cancer Care Alliance
Seattle, Washington
206.288.7222 • seattlecca.org
206.667.5000 • fredhutch.org

The Sidney Kimmel Comprehensive
Cancer Center at Johns Hopkins
Baltimore, Maryland
410.955.8964
hopkinsmedicine.org/kimmel_cancer_center

Robert H. Lurie Comprehensive
Cancer Center of Northwestern
University
Chicago, Illinois
866.587.4322 • cancer.northwestern.edu

Mayo Clinic Cancer Center
Phoenix/Scottsdale, Arizona
Jacksonville, Florida
Rochester, Minnesota
800.446.2279 • Arizona
904.953.0853 • Florida
507.538.3270 • Minnesota
mayoclinic.org/departments-centers/mayo-clinic-cancer-center

Memorial Sloan Kettering
Cancer Center
New York, New York
800.525.2225 • mskcc.org

Moffitt Cancer Center
Tampa, Florida
800.456.3434 • moffitt.org

The Ohio State University
Comprehensive Cancer Center -
James Cancer Hospital and
Solove Research Institute
Columbus, Ohio
800.293.5066 • cancer.osu.edu

O'Neal Comprehensive
Cancer Center at UAB
Birmingham, Alabama
800.822.0933 • uab.edu/onealcancercenter

Roswell Park Comprehensive
Cancer Center
Buffalo, New York
877.275.7724 • roswellpark.org

Siteman Cancer Center at Barnes-
Jewish Hospital and Washington
University School of Medicine
St. Louis, Missouri
800.600.3606 • siteman.wustl.edu

St. Jude Children's Research Hospital
The University of Tennessee
Health Science Center
Memphis, Tennessee
888.226.4343 • stjude.org
901.683.0055 • westclinic.com

Stanford Cancer Institute
Stanford, California
877.668.7535 • cancer.stanford.edu

UC San Diego Moores Cancer Center
La Jolla, California
858.657.7000 • cancer.ucsd.edu

UCLA Jonsson
Comprehensive Cancer Center
Los Angeles, California
310.825.5268 • cancer.ucla.edu

UCSF Helen Diller Family
Comprehensive Cancer Center
San Francisco, California
800.689.8273 • cancer.ucsf.edu

University of Colorado Cancer Center
Aurora, Colorado
720.848.0300 • coloradocancercenter.org

University of Michigan
Rogel Cancer Center
Ann Arbor, Michigan
800.865.1125 • rogelcancercenter.org

The University of Texas
MD Anderson Cancer Center
Houston, Texas
800.392.1611 • mdanderson.org

University of Wisconsin
Carbone Cancer Center
Madison, Wisconsin
608.265.1700 • uwhealth.org/cancer

UT Southwestern Simmons
Comprehensive Cancer Center
Dallas, Texas
214.648.3111 • utswmed.org/cancer

Vanderbilt-Ingram Cancer Center
Nashville, Tennessee
800.811.8480 • vicc.org

Yale Cancer Center/
Smilow Cancer Hospital
New Haven, Connecticut
855.4.SMILOW • yalecancercenter.org

Notes

Index

Made in the USA
Coppell, TX
10 May 2023

16633298R10024